How To Make A Homemade Lip Balm

30 DIY Quick Lip Balms Recipes for beginners

By April .K. Brown

Copyright

Table Of Content

Introduction

One of the easiest DIY products you can make at home and save a lot of money is the lip balm. The lips need nourishment, and the best thing is to pay attention to it, provides them with what they desire. The skin on our lips is super sensitive, and it is always affected by weather and lifestyle, which results in dry, peeling, and chapped lips.

Using natural ingredients helps you to get soft and luscious lips because it hydrates and help heal dry, chapped lips faster.

Making your lips balm is comfortable and healthy because you will know what your body is absorbing. The most interesting part of it is that you will enjoy experimenting with different recipes and make your choice ingredients. And also make it any flavor you want. In this book, there are lots of ingredients and recipes that will help you to make a fantastic natural homemade lip balm. The ingredients are available in your kitchen cabinet, so you don't need to go far.

This is an opportunity to be creative and create a signature lip balm. It is time to get to work; see you at the end.

Good luck

Chapter One

Some of the supplies needed

A. Heat-safe containers

They are in different shapes, sizes, and colors.

Choose the one that defines your work. Available in amazon store or you can still get them in your local stores

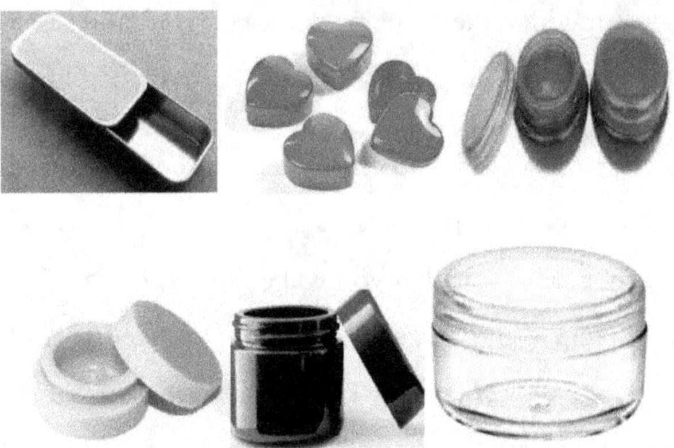

B. Digital scale

The digital scale is an accurate scale that will read to the nearest gram or 1/10 of an ounce. (Beam scale)

Or you can go on a digital kitchen scale.

When using a digital scale, place it on a hard surface for accuracy

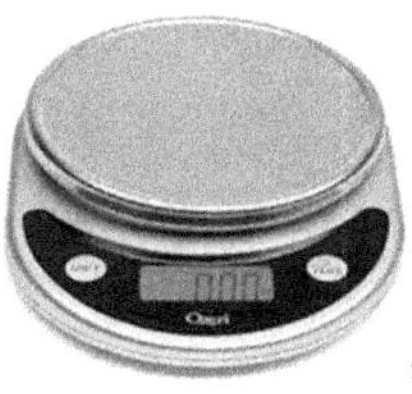

C. Spatula or spoon

You can use silicone or wood utensils.

It is advisable to use utensils with heat resistance up to 500 degrees.

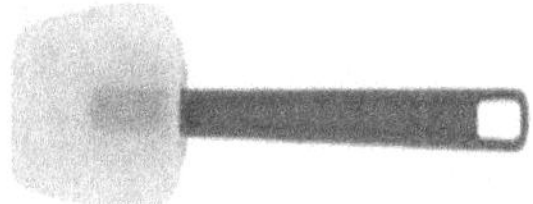

D. Hair net and gloves

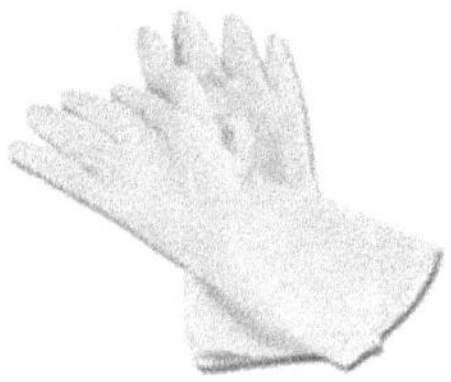

E. EMicrowave or double boiler

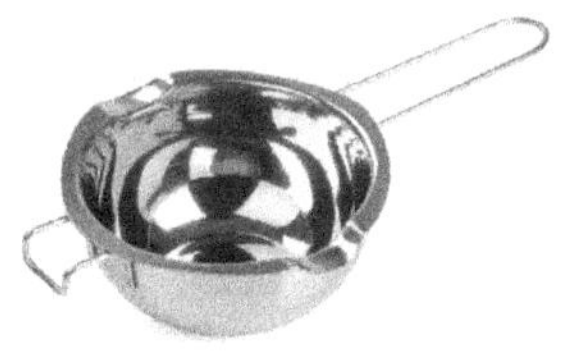

F. Plastic dropper

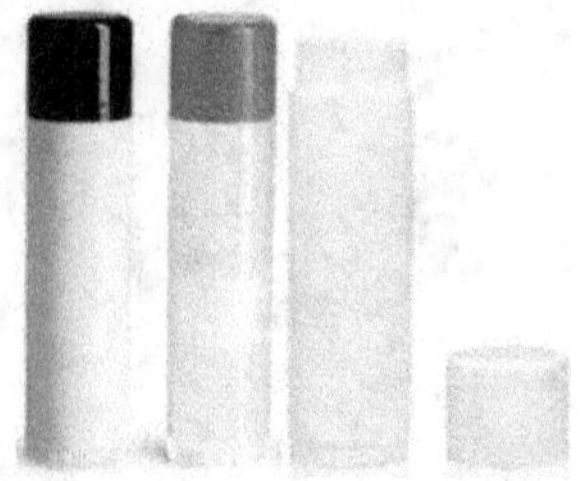

G. Measuring Spoon

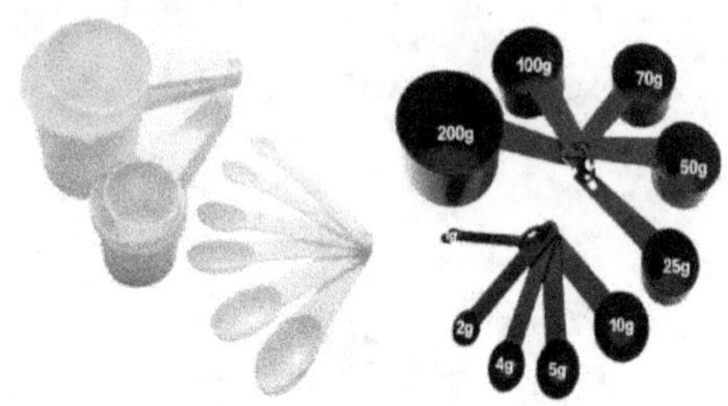

H. Measuring Cup

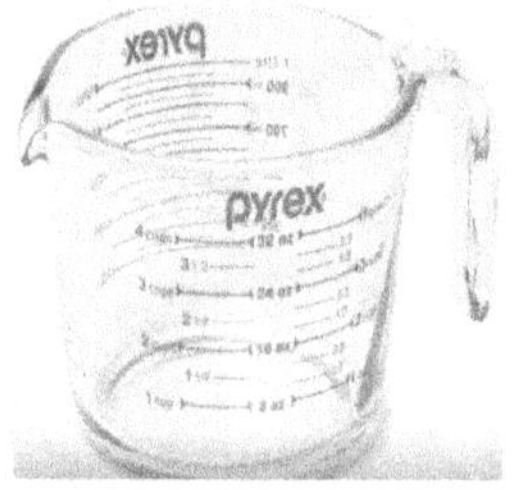

How to create a double boiler

Get a medium pot, fill it up to half with tap water, and place it on a stove. Get a smaller pot /measuring cup / safe heat container and place it inside the medium pot. Turn on stove to medium/ low heat, that how to create a double boiler. All

the ingredients you want to melt will be inside the smaller
pot.

Some Common Ingredients for homemade lip balm

1) Beeswax

The natural secretion from wax glands on the sides of the
body of a honey bee is known as beeswax. When the honey
bee feed with honey and huddle together to raise the
temperature of the cluster, it stimulates the production of
honeycomb.

To extract beeswax, boil honeycomb in water, the wax will
settle on top, skim it off the top, which becomes your
beeswax. It comes in different colors like yellow, white, and
brown. Beeswax has a natural aroma because of the fragrance
of honey embedded in it. Beeswax natural hydrating
properties help retain natural skin moisture when in contact
with human skin.

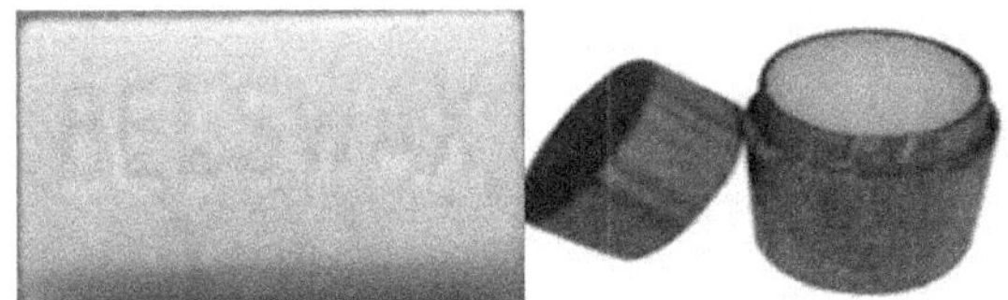

2) Shea butter

Shea butter is extracted from a seed fat that comes from the
Shea tree found in East and west tropical Africa. The two oily

kernels are removed from the seed and grounded into a powder and then boil in water. The oil/ butter rise to the top of the water and become solid. 100 percent pure, unrefined, raw shea butter is full of all-natural vitamin A,

Shea butter, because of its moisturizing and hydrating property it provides immediate softness and smoothness when applied to the skin.

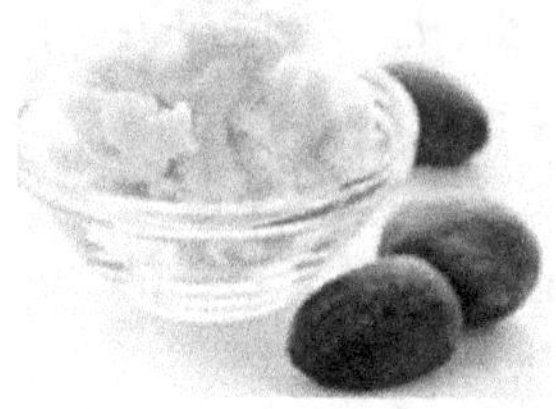

3) Extra-virgin coconut oil

It is the grade of coconut oil that is unrefined, which contains healthy MCTs (medium- chain triglycerides) & lauric acid.

This oil is extracted directly from the fresh meat of coconut kernels.

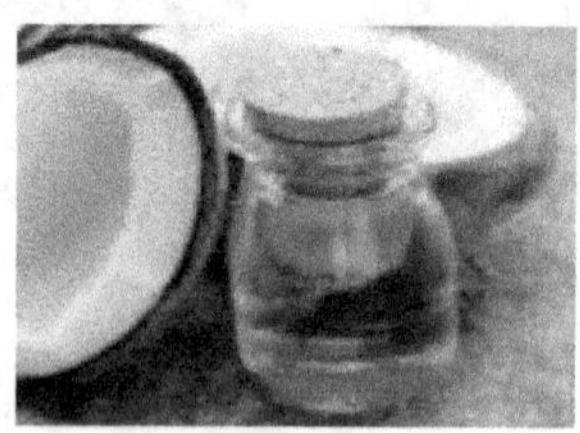

4) Cocoa Butter

Cocoa butter, a natural ingredient rich in fats, is extracted from the cocoa beans. It has a sweet aroma and velvety in texture. It also contains Vitamins E and omega three unsaturated fats. It is good for chapped lips because it keeps it hydrated.

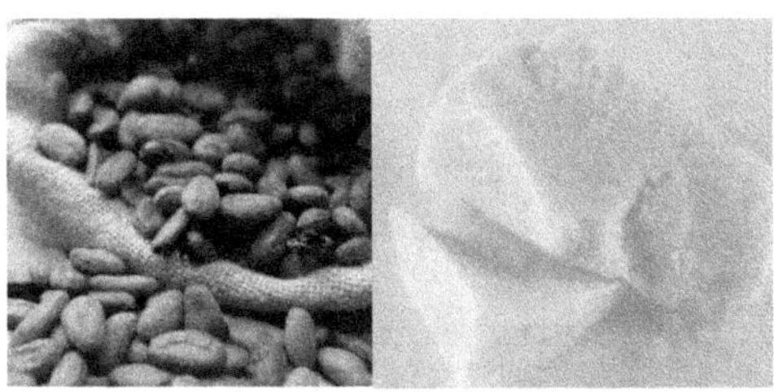

5) Mango Butter

Mango butter is a hugely beneficial ingredient for lip balms. Its soft creamy texture makes it easy to use and well absorbed by the skin. The mango butter rejuvenated the skin, treat dry skin, and provide long-lasting emollience.

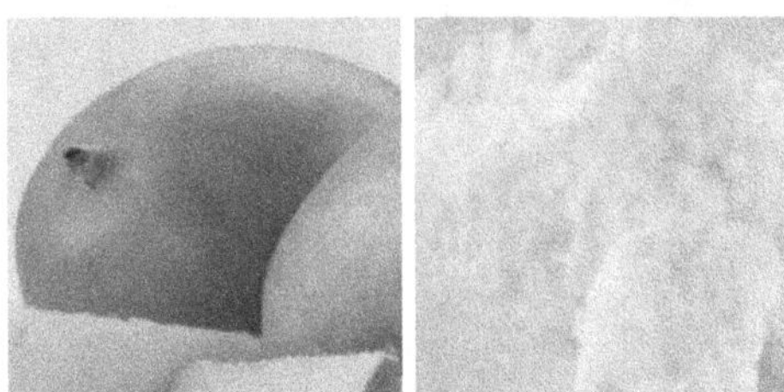

6) Olive oil

Olive oil, a Mediterranean diet, is full of anti-aging antioxidants. A natural moisturizer, skin softener, skin healer and prevents premature aging of the skin.

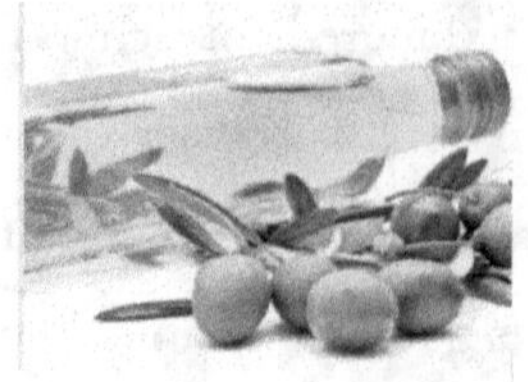

7) Rosehip seed oil

Rosehip oil is oil extracted from the hip of a specific variety of rose known as "Rosa canina" The term hip is defined as the leftover fruit after a rose has bloomed and the petals withered. The oil is rich in essentials fatty acids and Vitamins A, C, and E. it is suitable for any skin and easily absorbed by the skin.

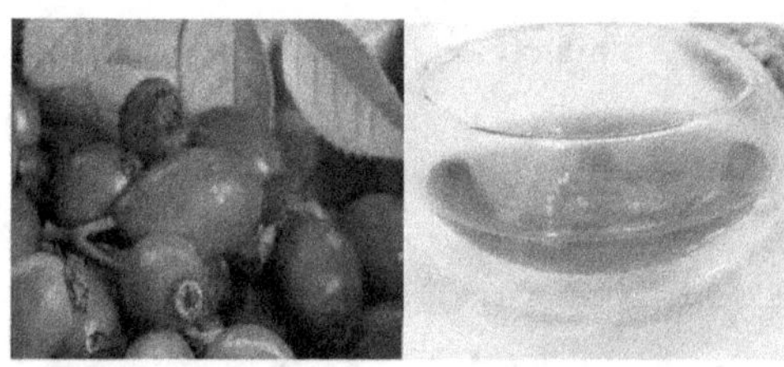

8) Grape seed oil

Grape seed oil, a byproduct of the winemaking process, is extracted from the seeds of the pressed grapes. It has anti-inflammatory, antimicrobial, and antioxidant properties. The oil is rich in omega chain fatty acids and Vitamin E, which made it a popular, topical skin treatment.

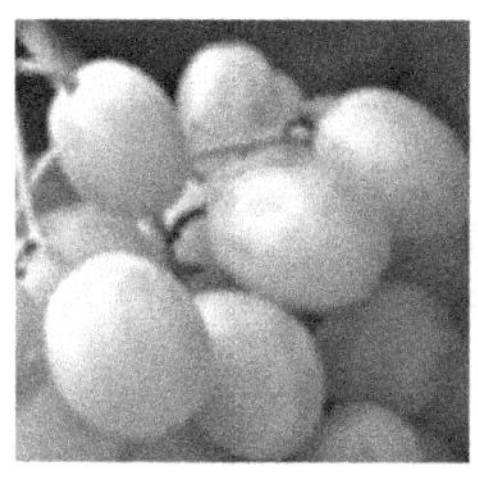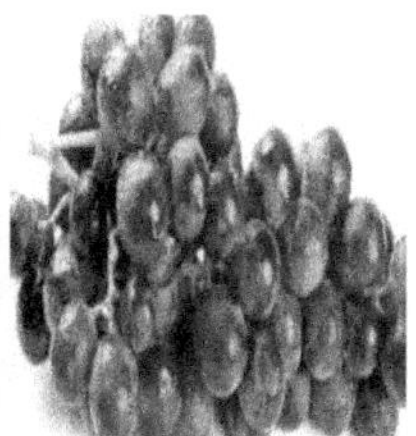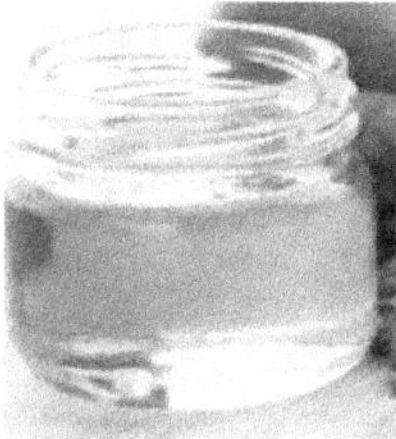

9) Avocado oil

Avocado oil is carrier oil that is rich with omega-three fatty acids and vitamins A, D, and E. when used on the lips, it moisturizes and nourishes it.

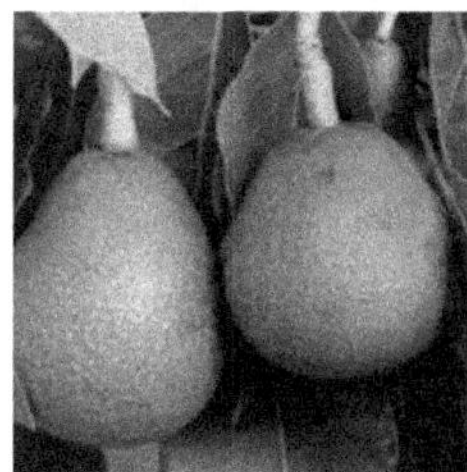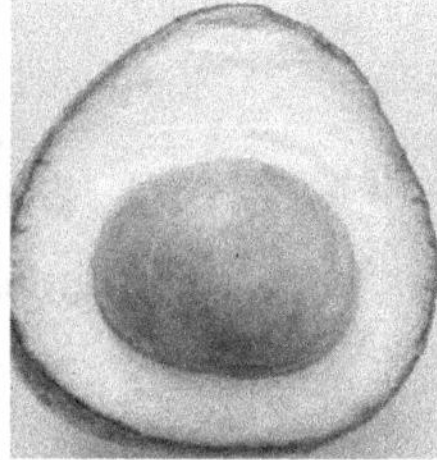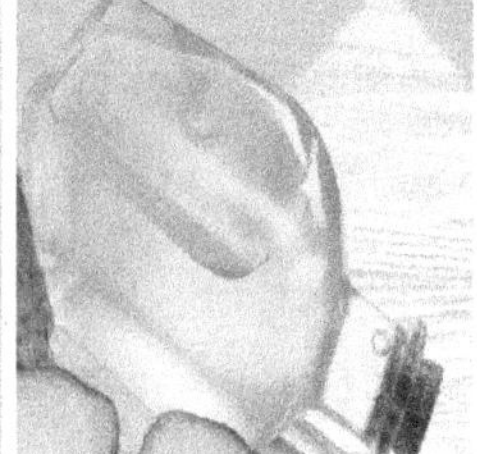

10) Lanolin Oil

Lanolin oil is secretion that comes out from sheepskin (sebaceous glands). The extraction process is performed on **the wool of the sheep after the sheep have been sheared**. It causes no harm to the sheep. It is emollient oil that helps soothe dry or dehydrated lips and fixed chapped lips.

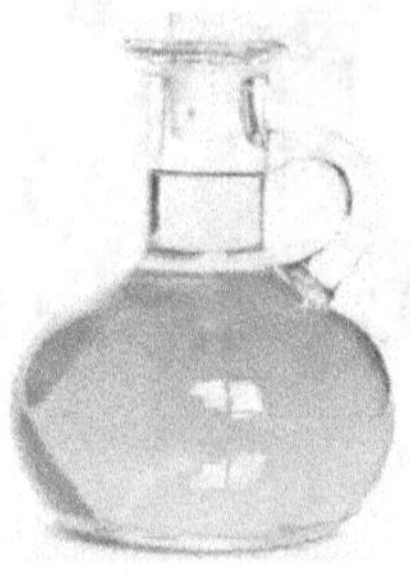

11) Almond oil

Almond oil, an extract from the edible seeds of the almond tree called Prunus dulcis. The process of extraction, which is pressing raw almonds without using high temperatures or chemical agents, retains most of its nutrients. Almond oil has been customarily used in many ways on the skin because of its anti-inflammatory, emollient, immunity-boosting, and sclerosant properties.

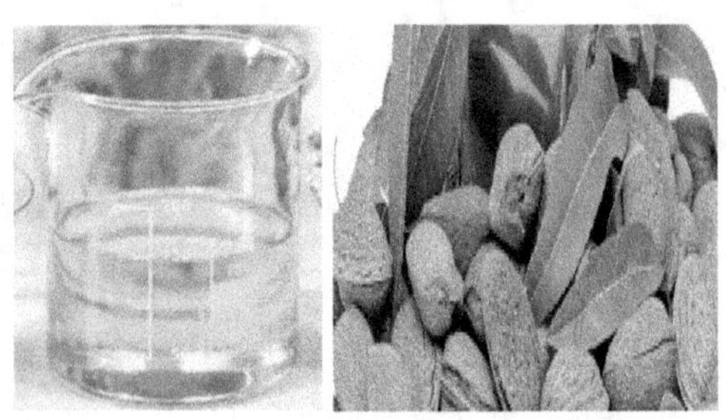

Chapter Two

Part one Recipes

Beeswax lip balm

<u>**Ingredients**</u>

1. 1 tablespoon grated beeswax

2. 1 tablespoon extra-virgin coconut oil

3. A little dash of organic raw honey

4. 2 capsules of vitamin E

<u>**Procedure**</u>

Melt down the beeswax in a double boiler and once melted, add the measured coconut oil and honey.

Or

Put a heat-safe bowl carefully on top of a pot of boiling water over medium-low heat. Add the beeswax, shea butter, and honey inside the heat-safe bowl.

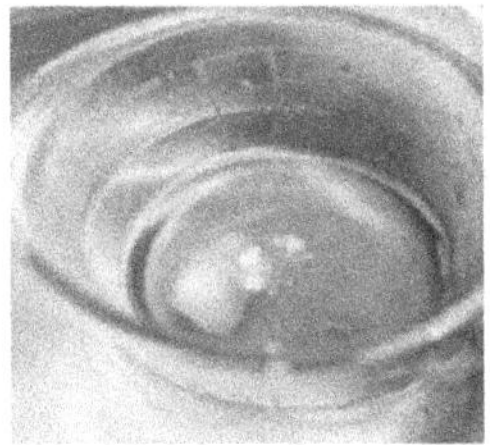

Heat for about 10 -15 minutes until the ingredients are completely melted.

Use a spatula to blend the ingredients.

Remove from heat and add two capsules of vitamin E oil.

Transfer the product into a glass cup or a measuring cup with a spout.

From the measuring cup, pour the finished product into a tin or empty lip balm tubes and fill up to the brim.

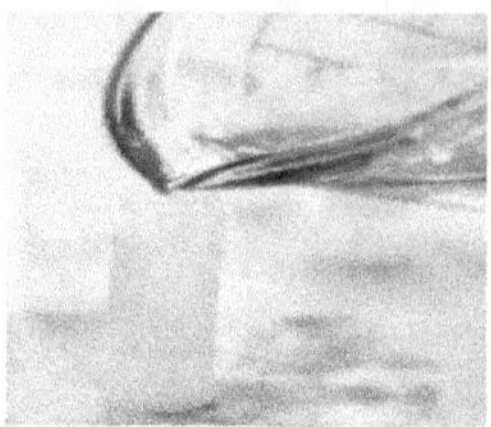

Allow the mixture to cool for sometimes say 30 minutes before placing a cap on top.

Ready for use

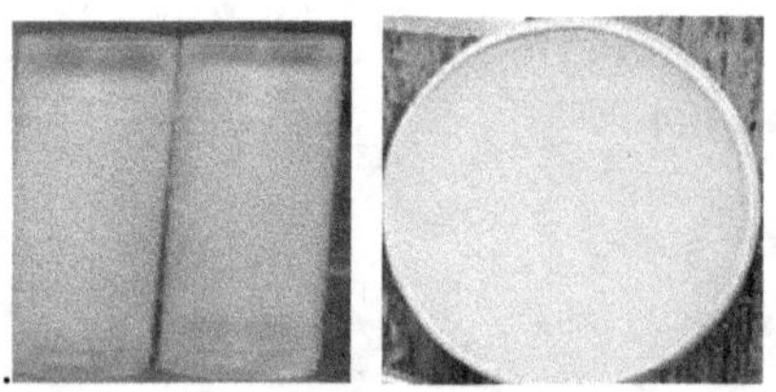

Pink Grapefruit Lip Balm

Ingredients

1 tablespoon of coconut oil

1 tablespoon of white beeswax pellets

1 tablespoon of sweet almond oil

1 inch piece of red lip balm (optional for color)

10 drop of grapefruit essential oil

Procedure

In a double boiler, meltdown all the ingredients for the balm.

Or

Put a heat - safe bowl carefully on the pot of simmering water over medium -low heat. Add all the ingredients inside the heat - safe bowl.

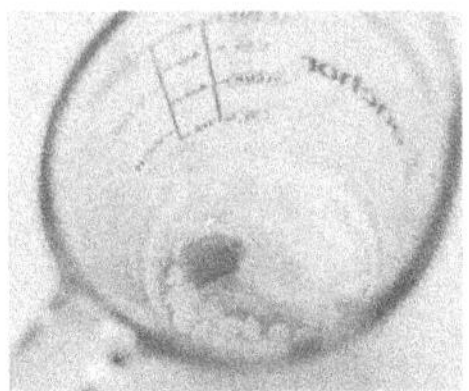

Once the ingredients got melted, blend thoroughly with a spatula.

Immediately add several drops of grapefruit essential oil for flavor and scent.

Transfer the mixture into a glass cup or a measuring cup with a spout.

From the measuring cup, pour the finished product into a tin or empty lip balm tubes and fill up to the brim.

Or

You can get a large syringe to fill the container or empty lip balm carefully.

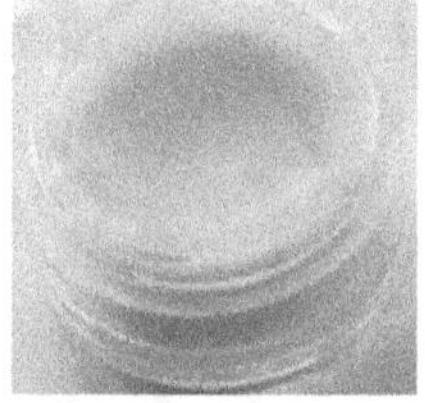

Mint Chocolate lip balm

Ingredients

For 10 empty lip balm tools

2 tablespoon of Beeswax pellets

2 tablespoon of Organic Coconut Oil

1/2 teaspoon grated Cocoa Butter

2 tablespoon sweet almond oil

4 drops of peppermint essential oil

2 Chocolate Chips

Procedure.

In a heat-safe bowl, add the beeswax pellets and Chocolate Chips.

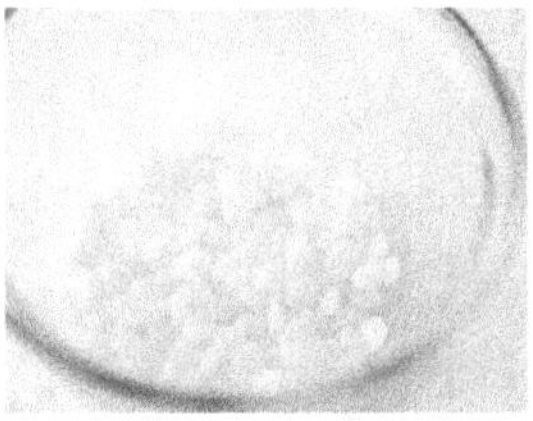

Place on a double boiler and allow it to melt

Once melted remove it from the heat and melt cocoa butter

Place back in the heat, add coconut oil and stir all using spatula until the mixture becomes smooth.

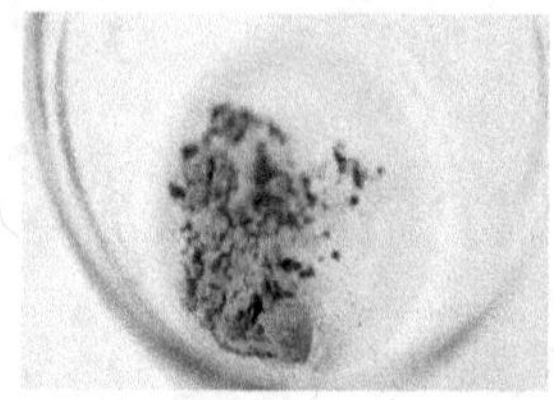

Bring down and add sweet almond oil and four drops of peppermint oil.

Transfer the mixture into a glass cup or a measuring cup with a spout.

From the measuring cup, pour the finished product into a tin or empty lip balm tubes and fill up to the brim.

Or

You can get a large syringe to fill the container or empty lip balm carefully.

Let it sit for at least 15 minutes, depending on the weather.

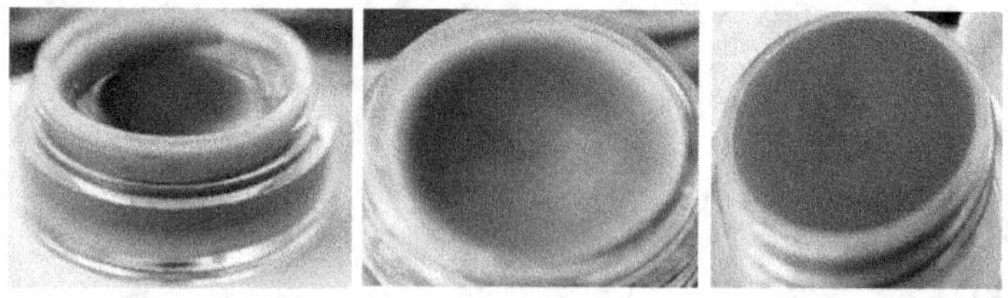

Coconut oil lip balm

Ingredients

2 teaspoon virgin coconut oil

2 teaspoon petroleum jelly

Procedure

In a heat-safe bowl, add the virgin coconut oil and petroleum jelly.

Place on a double boiler and allow it to melt

Once melted stir thoroughly with a spatula

Remove from heat

Transfer the mixture into a glass cup or a measuring cup with a spout.

From the measuring cup pour the finished product into a tin or empty lip balm tubes and fill up to the brim.

Freeze for 20 to 30 minutes

Coconut oil and Aloe Vera

Ingredients

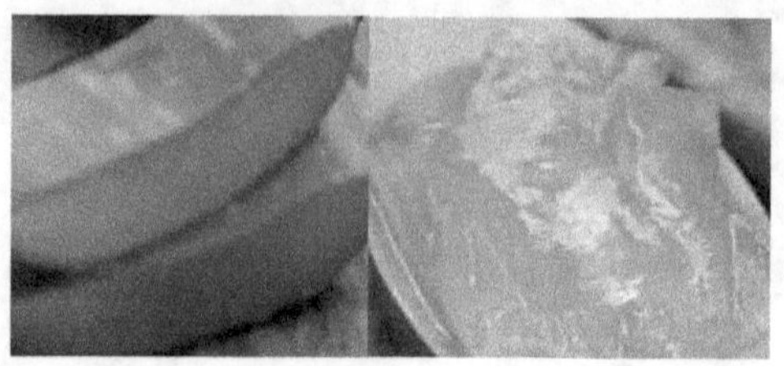

2 tablespoon of coconut oil

1 tablespoon of carnauba wax

2 teaspoon of aloe Vera gel (extracted from the aloe vera stick).

Procedure

In a heat-safe bowl, add the virgin coconut oil and Carnauba wax.

Place on a double boiler and allow it to melt

Once melted, bring it down and add aloe vera gel.

Mix thoroughly and pour the mixture into lip balm container and allow it to set.

Coconut oil and olive balm

Ingredients

2 tablespoon of coconut oil

2 tablespoon of carnauba wax

2 tablespoon of olive oil

Procedure

In a heat- safe bowl, add the virgin coconut oil, Carnauba wax and olive oil.

Place on a double boiler and allow it to melt.

Once melted, bring it down and add aloe vera gel.

Mix thoroughly and pour the mixture into lip balm container and allow it to set.

Coconut oil and shea butter oil

Ingredients

2 tablespoon of coconut oil

2 tablespoon of carnauba wax

2 tablespoon of shea butter

Procedure

In a heat -safe bowl, add the virgin coconut oil, Carnauba wax and shea butter.

Place on a double boiler and allow it to melt.

Once melted, bring it down.

Mix thoroughly and pour the mixture into lip balm container and allow it to set. Or you can put inside a fridge.

You can also try these coconut oil recipes.

Coconut oil and red palm fruit oil
Ingredients

2 tablespoon of coconut oil

2 teaspoon of red palm fruit oil.

Follow the normal procedure of coconut oil recipes.

Coconut oil and lavender lip balm
Ingredients

3 tablespoons of coconut oil

2 tablespoon of carnauba wax

20 drops of lavender essential oil

Same procedure as above.

Lemonade lip balm

Ingredients

2 tablespoon of coconut oil

2 tablespoon of Beeswax

1 tablespoon of cocoa butter

1 tablespoon of shea butter

30 drops of doTerra lemon essential oil

Procedure

Add shea butter, virgin coconut oil, beeswax and cocoa butter in a heat - safe bowl.

Place on a double boiler and allow it to melt.

Once melted, bring it down.

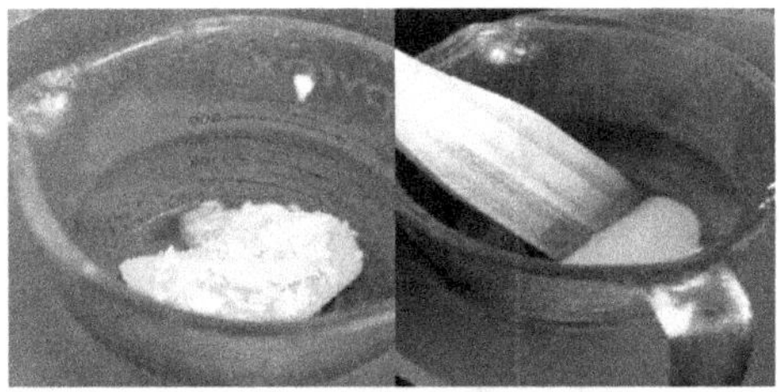

Stir in the lemon essential oil drop by drop until you reach your desired taste.

Immediately pour the mixture into a measuring cup and from there fill in the tubes or containers.

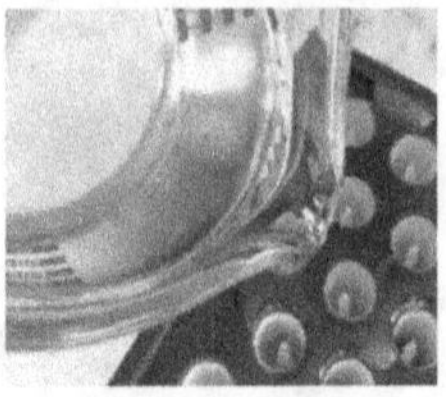

Allow to cool for sometimes before use.

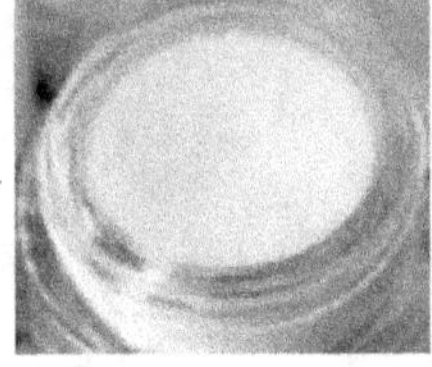

Pink Lemonade

Ingredients

1/2 cup of sweet almond oil

4 teaspoon of magenta or red beet powder

1 ounce beeswax

1/2 teaspoon vitamin E

30 drop of lemons essential oil

Procedure

Put all the ingredients in a heat safe bowel except essential oil.

Place on a double boiler and allow it to melt over medium heat. Stir the mixture severally until there are no clumps of beetroot left.

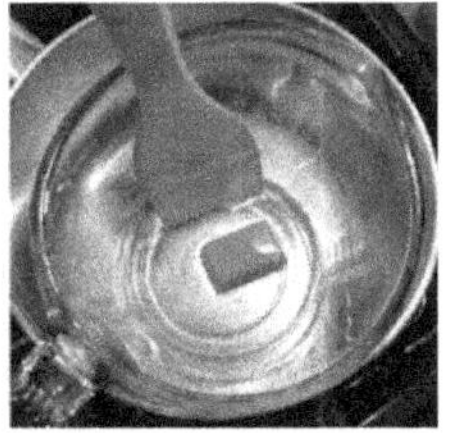

Bring down from the heat and add essential oil to the mix.

Stir thoroughly and pour the mix immediately inside the tubes or container.

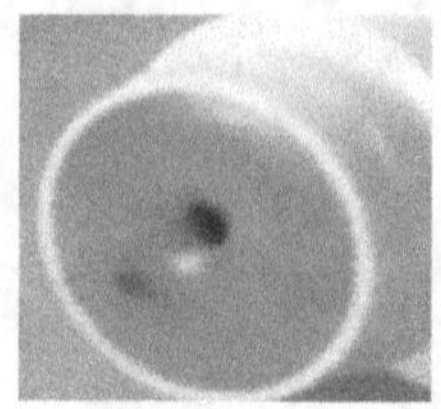

Raspberry and lemon lip balm

Ingredients

2 teaspoons of raspberry gelatin mix

2 tablespoons of virgin coconut oil

3-4 drops of lemon essential oil

Procedure

In a double boiler, melt the coconut oil and when it is almost done, add the raspberry gelatin. Mix the two ingredients thoroughly until the gelatin melts.

You will observe that the oil has a deep raspberry color.

Or

Put a heat - safe bowl carefully on top of a pot of boiling water over medium - low heat. Add the coconut oil and raspberry gelatin inside the heat - safe bowl.

Allow the ingredients to melt and mix thoroughly.

Bring down from the heat

Immediately add the lemon essential oil and continuously stir until everything mixed properly.

Transfer the mixture into a measuring cup.

From the measuring cup pour the mixture in the lip balm container, tubes or any container of your choice.

Allow to cool, say about 20- 30 minutes or place in a refrigerator until it hardens.

Start using immediately

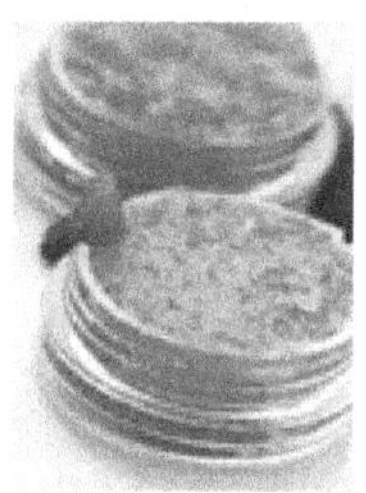

Pure Essential oil Lip Balm

Ingredients

1 tablespoon of beeswax beads

3 tablespoon of coconut oil or your favorite carrier oil

1 teaspoon of beetroot powder

5 drops of vitamin E oil

2 drop of rosemary essential oil

3 drops of peppermint essential oil

4 drops of Lemon essential oil

Procedure

In a glass measuring cup or heat-safe bowl, add the coconut oil, beeswax beads.

Put inside a microwave to melt

Or

Put the heat safe bowl carefully on a pot of simmering water over medium-low heat.

Allow it to melt. Melting time depends on the quantity you are melting.'

This quantity took about 90 seconds to melt completely.

Once melted, mix thoroughly

Bring down from the heat.

Add all the Essential oil and mix well

To give it a color, add a little quantity of beetroot powder and stir well until no lumps are seen.

Immediately pour inside the lip balm tubes, lip balm container, or any container of your choice.

Allow to cool, or you can put in a refrigerator to harden.

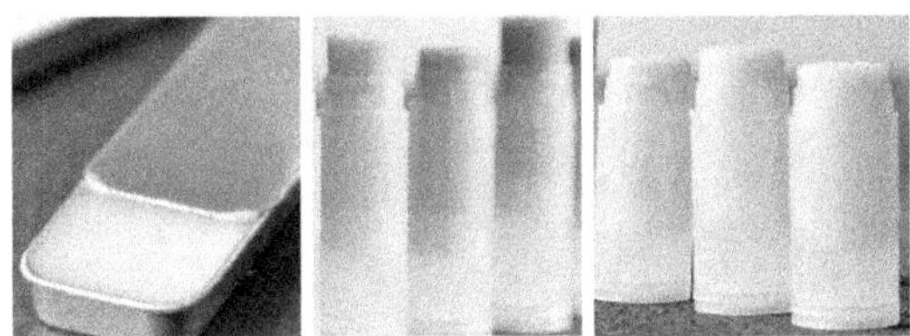

Lavender Honey Lip Balm

(For 12 lip balm tubes)

Ingredients

2 Tablespoon of coconut oil

1 Tablespoon of shea butter

1/2 Teaspoon of raw honey

1 Tablespoon of sweet almond

2 Tablespoon of Beeswax

15 drops of lavender essential oil

5 drops of frankincense essential oil

Procedure

In a heat-safe bowl, add the coconut oil, Shea butter, honey, and beeswax.

Gently place on a pot of simmering water over medium-low heat.

Stir continually until the ingredients melt. Once melted, remove from heat and stir in the sweet almond, lavender essential oil ad frankincense essential oil.

To avoid the setting of the oil, pour the mixture immediately inside the measuring cup. From the measuring cup, transfer the mixture to the lip balm tubes or containers.

Allow hardening

Ready for use

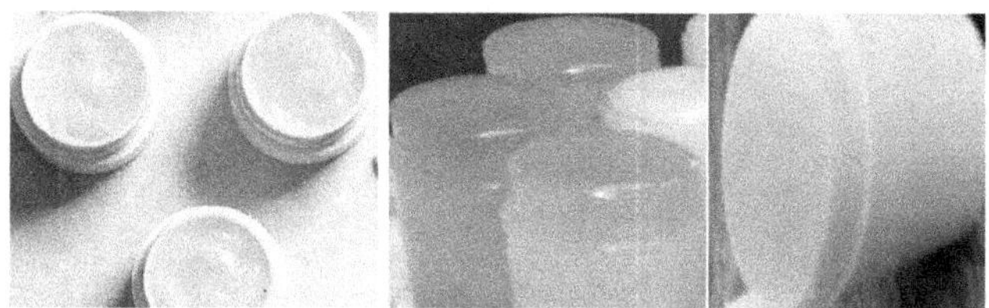

Rose Lip Balm

Ingredients

1 tablespoon of beeswax

1/2 tablespoon of castor oil

3 tablespoons of rose-infused oil (extracted from dried rose petal)

1 teaspoon of vanilla extract

1 tablespoon of cocoa butter

1/4 teaspoon of powered alkanet root

4 – 5 drops of rose essential oil

Procedure

In a heat-safe bowl (Put the heat-safe bowl carefully on a pot of simmering water over medium-low heat).

First melt the beeswax then add the castor oil, cocoa butter, and rose-infused oil.

Once melted, add the alkanet root powder and stir thoroughly to make sure there is no lump.

Bring down from the heat

Add vanilla extract and rose essential oil for some fragrance.

Pour the mixture inside a lip balm containers or tubes and allow to set.

Store for six months

How to extract oil from dried rose petal

Get a jar, preferably glass jar and fill it 3/4 with dried rose petals,(Chose a jar that will contain the quantity of dried rose petal that you have).

Cover with oil like olive oil or sunflower for lip balm.

Place the jar gently in a pan of warm water and heat slowly over simmering heat. Reduce the heat to the minimum and allow the jar to sit in the heated water for one to two hours,

Remove from heat and strain the oil.

The oil is now ready for use.

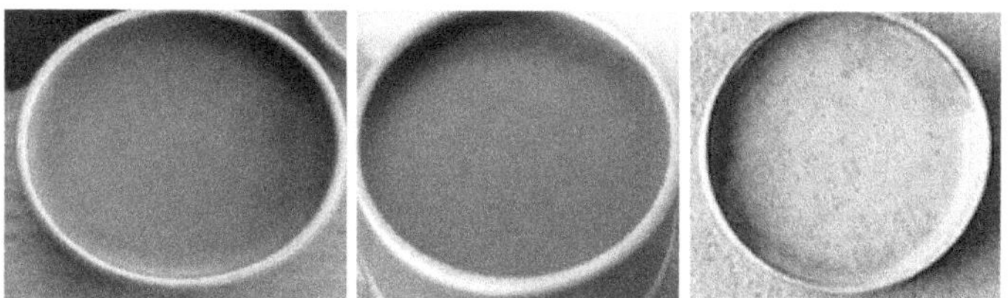

Chapter Three

Part Two Recipes

Honey and hemp lip balm

Ingredients

15 g of beeswax

1 g of carnauba wax

10 g of cocoa butter

5 g of shea butter

4 teaspoon of almond oil

1 teaspoon of hemp oil

2 teaspoon of Manuka honey (purchase from Amazon or your local store).

8 drops of citrus essential oil

Procedure

In a heat-safe bowl add the beeswax, carnauba wax, cocoa butter, shea butter, and Almond oil.

Gently place on a pot of simmering water over medium-low heat.

Stir continually until the ingredients melt.

Add hemp oil, honey, and citrus essential oil in the mixture stir until it turns into a liquid consistency.

Remove from heat

Blend using a milk frother.

Once the mixtures reach medium-thick consistency, pour inside a lip balm containers or tubes and allow to cool for sometimes.

Store for six months

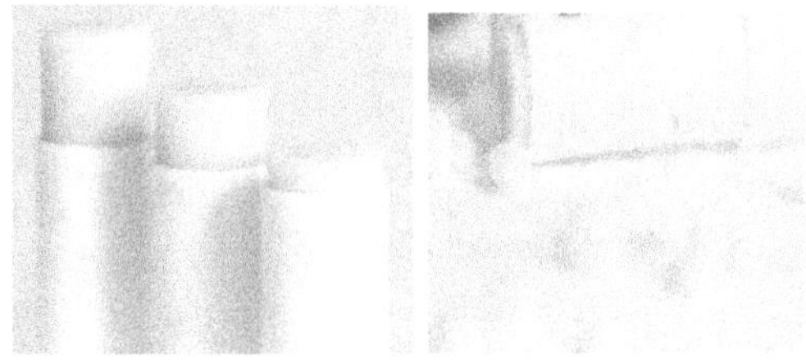

Ultra healing lip balm

For 20 lip balm tubes

This is specifically to cure dried, cracked, and chapped lips.

Ingredients

2 teaspoons of sweet almond oil

1 teaspoon of jojoba oil

1 teaspoon of mango butter

1 teaspoon of beeswax

3 drops of lavender essential oil

3 drops of lime/lemon/orange essential

2 drops of vitamin E

2 drops of d-panthenol (optional)

Procedure

In a heat-safe bowl put the beeswax, mango butter, jojoba oil, and sweet almond oil.

Gently place on a pot of simmering water over medium-low heat.

Stir continually until the ingredients melt.

Remove from the heat and stir in lavender essential oil, Vitamin E, and lime essential oil.

You can also add d-panthenol if you desire.

Whisk together all the ingredients using egg whisker.

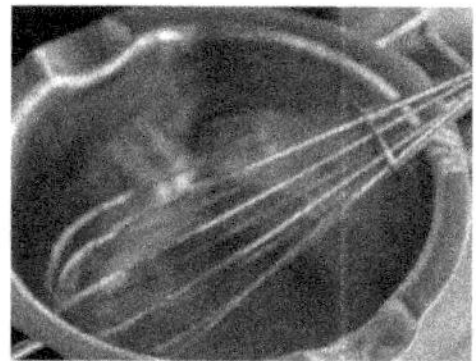

Transfer the mixture into a measuring cup, from there pour in the lip balm tubes or lips balm container or any container of your choice.

Allow to cool for sometimes.

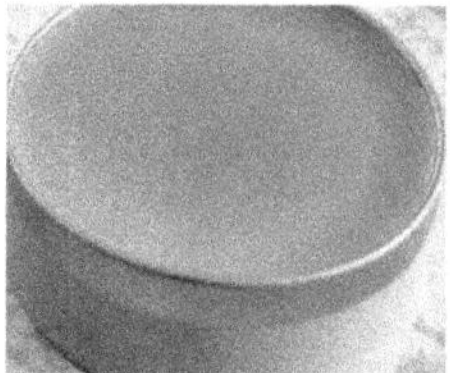 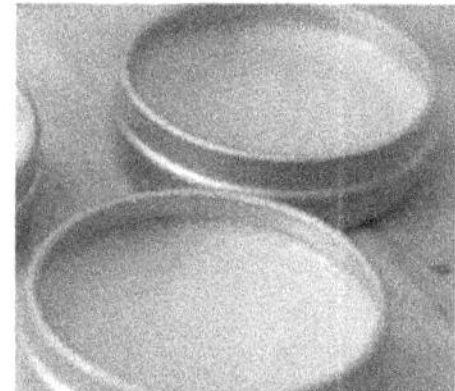

Sweet orange and calendula soothing lip balm

Ingredients

14 g of organic natural beeswax beads

7 g of organic cocoa butter

14 g of organic shea butter

22 g of organic Brazil Nut oil

3 g of organic calendula oil extract

3 g of organic golden jojoba oil

10 drops of organic sweet orange essential oil

Procedure

In a heat-safe bowl, combine the beeswax, cocoa butter, and shea butter.

Gently place on a pot of simmering water over medium-low heat.

Stir continually until the ingredients melt.

Remove the bowl from heat

Add organic Brazil nut oil, calendula oil, and sweet orange Essential oil to the mixture and stir thoroughly.

Transfer into the lip balm tubes or lip balm containers. Allow to cool.

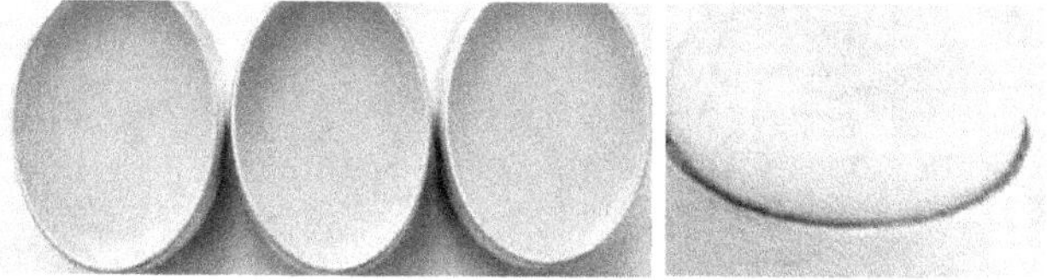

Shea butter lip balm

Ingredients

1 tablespoon of shea butter

1 tablespoon of beeswax

1 teaspoon raw honey

1 tablespoon of raw organic coconut oil

15 drops of lemon balm essential oil

5 drops roman chamomile essential oil

3-5 drops of lavender essential oil

2–4 drops of orange essential oil

Procedure

Combine shea butter, beeswax, and organic coconut oil and melt in a double boiler.

Stir continually until the ingredients melt.

Once melted turn off the stove

Add raw honey and all the essential oil.

Whisk all together until well blended.

Pour the mixture inside a measuring cup.

Transfer from the measuring cup to lip balm containers or lip balms tubes.

All to cool or put in the refrigerator to harden

Enjoy

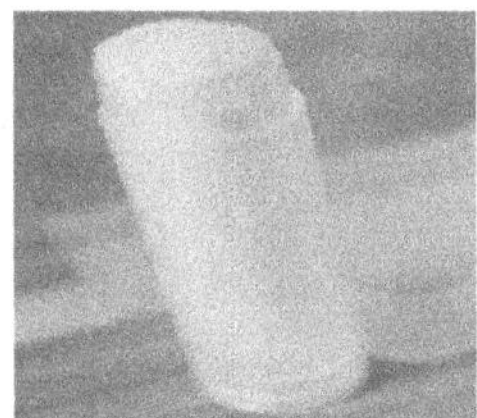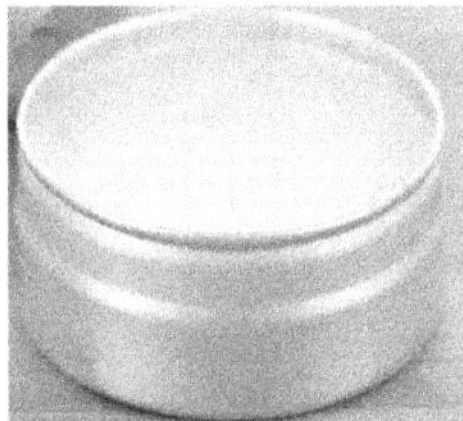

Nutmeg & mandarin lip balm

Ingredients

1 tablespoon plus 1 teaspoon of beeswax

1 tablespoon of organic mango butter

2 tablespoon of organic sunflower

1 tablespoon of organic olive oil

15 drops of organic mandarin essential oil

5 drops of organic nutmeg essential oil

2 drops of vitamin E oil

Procedure

In a heat-safe bowl put the beeswax, mango butter, sunflower oil, and organic olive oil.

Gently place on a pot of simmering water over medium-low heat.

Stir continually until the ingredients melt.

Remove from the heat and stir in the essential oils and Vitamin E oil.

Pour the mixture immediately in lip balm containers or lip balm tubes.

Put in the refrigerator to harden

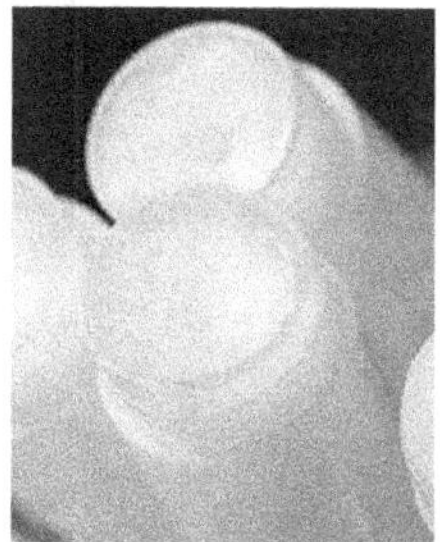

45

Lemon zest Recipes

Ingredients

1 tablespoon of Vaseline

1 teaspoon of lemon juice

1 teaspoon of honey

Procedure

In a glass measuring cup or heat-safe bowl, put the Vaseline

Put inside a microwave to melt

Once melted, add the lemon juice and honey, blend by mixing with a milk frother or egg whisk.

Pour the mixtures in a lip balm container and allow to cool

Kool-Aid lip balm

Recipes 1

Ingredients

1 sachet of kool-Aid

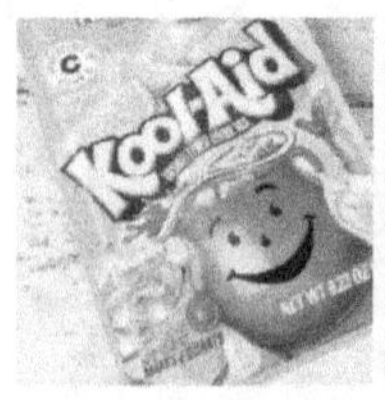
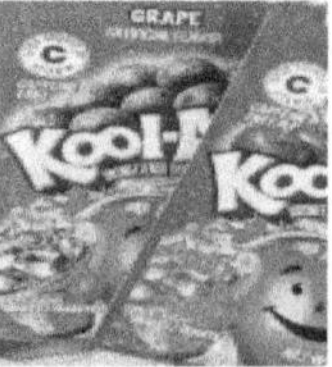

1 teaspoon of sugar (optional)

1 teaspoon of water

1 tablespoon of organic coconut oil

Procedure

In a measuring cup or glass bowl, pour the entire kool-aid sachet.

Add sugar.

Add a teaspoon of water to dissolve the mix.

Add organic cocoa nut oil to the mixture and stir till they are properly blended.

From the measuring cup, transfer the mixture to the lip balm tubes or lip balm containers.

Allow to set in a refrigerator.

Recipes 2

Ingredients

1 tablespoon of petroleum jelly

1 sachet of kool Aid

Procedure

In a double boiler melt the petroleum jelly

Bring down from heat and stir in one sachet of kool Aid.

Mix the ingredients thoroughly until you get an excellent consistency.

Pour inside lip balm container and allow to set

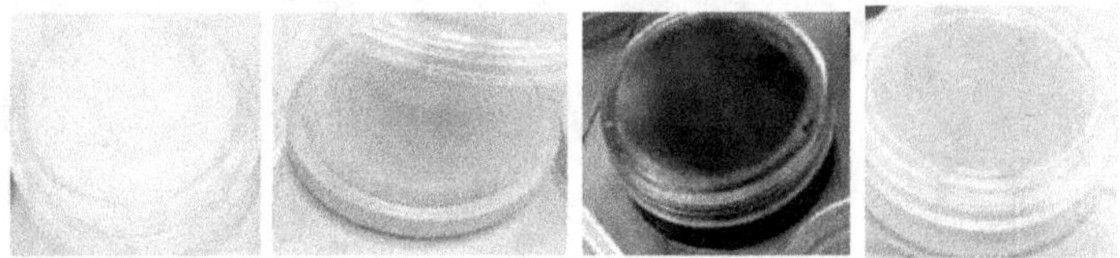

Beetroot lip balm

<u>**Recipes 1**</u>

Ingredients

Farm fresh beetroot

1 teaspoon of Coconut oil

Procedure

Gently wash the beetroot under running water to remove all the dirt.

With a sharp knife peel off the hard outer layer of the beetroot

Chop the beetroot into small sizes.

Pour inside a food processor and grind until the beetroot is grounded, leaving a watery residue.

Note: do not add water during grinding to avoid diluting the consistency of the color

Strain the grounded beetroot with a fine strainer to get the juice.

Transfer the juice inside a clean container.

Add coconut oil inside the juice and stir to blend

Pour in a lip balm tubes or empty lip balm container

Place the containers inside the refrigerator to set.

Your lip balm is ready for use.

Recipes 2

3g of beeswax

6 g of virgin coconut oil

16 g of castor oil

10 g of jojoba oil

1 g of Vitamin E oil

4 g of vegetable glycerin

1 teaspoon of beetroot powder

Procedure

In a double boiler combine and melt the beeswax and the oil

Stir in the vegetable glycerin and the beetroot extract/power. Bring down from the heat.

Mix the ingredients thoroughly until they are well blended. Allow the cream to cool to a thick mixture. Whisk together again until you have a thick maroon mixture.

Scoop and put it in a lip balm container.

Your lip balm is ready.

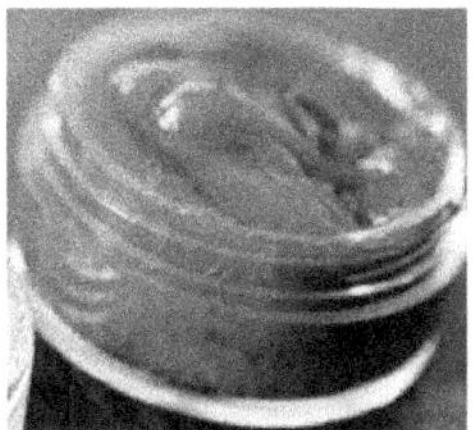

Honey hippie

Ingredients

1 teaspoon of coconut oil

1 teaspoon of olive oil

1 teaspoon of lanolin

1 teaspoon shea butter

1 teaspoon honey

1 teaspoon of beeswax pastilles

Procedure

Melt the oils and beeswax pastilles in double boilers

Remove from heat and whisk in the honey.

Transfer the mixture to measuring cup from there pours into lip balm tubes, lip balm containers.

Allow to cool or put in a refrigerator to set.

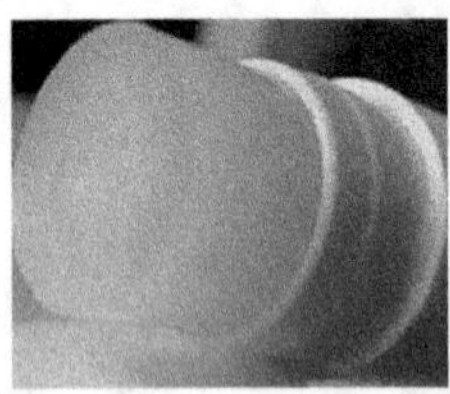

Banana Lip Balm

Ingredients

1 tablespoon of coconut oil

1 tablespoon of Beeswax

1/2 tablespoon of shea butter

1/2 tablespoon of cocoa butter

4 -6 drops of Banana Cream flavor oil

Procedure

Combine and melt the ingredients in a double boiler over medium heat.

Stir continuously and remove from heat

Stir in the banana flavor gradually until you reach your desired flavor

Allow to cool for about 30 minutes or more.

Enjoy.

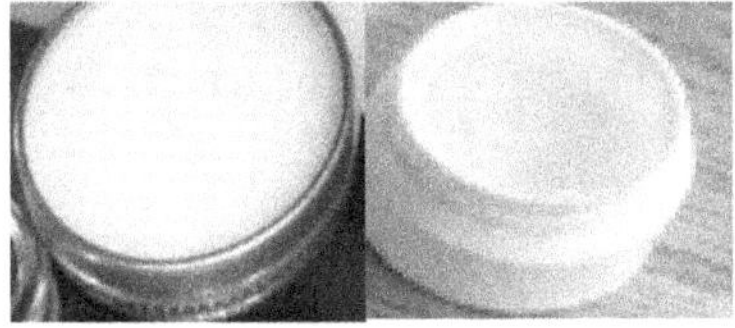

Lemon rosemary Lip Balm

Ingredients

1 teaspoon of almond oil

2 tablespoon of beeswax beads

1 teaspoon of vitamin E oil

15 drops lemon of essential oil

15 drops of rosemary essential oil

1 tablespoon of castor oil

Procedure

Melt the beeswax oil and almond oils in a double boiler over medium heat.

Stir the ingredients continuously until they are melted.

Remove from heat

Stir in Vitamin E oil, lemon, and rosemary essentials oils.

Mix thoroughly until well blended.

Pour the mixture in a measuring cup, from there pour to the lip balm tubes, container.

Allow to cool for sometime

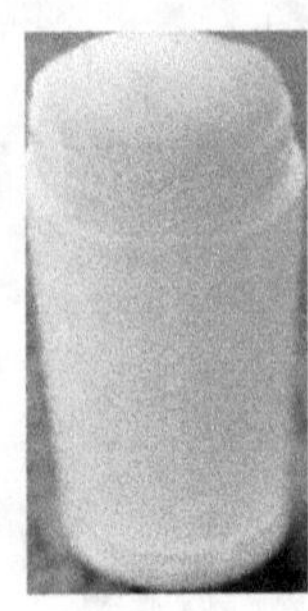

Lime lip balm

Ingredients

1 tablespoon coconut oil

1 teaspoon of cocoa butter

1 teaspoon of almond oil

1 teaspoon of beeswax.

5 to 10 drops of pure lime essential oil

Procedure

Melt the cocoa butter, coconut oil, beeswax and almond oil in a double boiler over medium heat.

Stir the ingredients continuously until they are melted.

Remove from heat. Stir in lime essentials oil.

Transfer the mixture to measuring cup and from there pours inside lip balm tubes or container.

Allow to cool before use

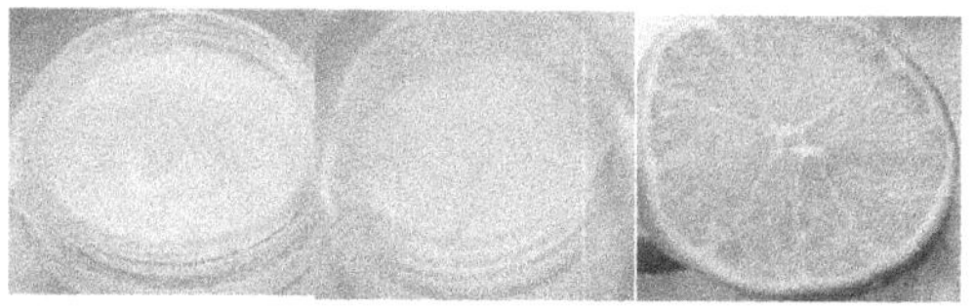

Anti-aging lip balm

Ingredients

1 tablespoon of cocoa butter

2 tablespoon of beeswax

5 drops of carrot seed essential oil

1 tablespoon of Coconut oil

1 drop of frankincense essential oil

3 drops of peppermint essential oil

1 tablespoon of Rosehip seed oil

Procedure

In a double boiler, combine and melt the beeswax, coconut butter, and coconut oil over medium heat; stir till the entire ingredients are melted.

Remove from heat and allow to cool for say 2 minutes.

Stir in all the essential oils until they are well blended.

Transfer to the measuring cup. Pour inside lip balm tubes or containers.

Put in a refrigerator to harden or allow to cool for half an hour.

Cherry lip

Ingredients

For 15 lip balm tubes

2 tablespoon of avocado oil

4 tablespoon coconut oil

2 tablespoon beeswax

2-3 drops of flavor oil

1 ml of vitamin E oil

Pinch of safe lip mica

Procedure

In a double boiler, combine the avocado, beeswax, and coconut oil and melt over medium heat; stir till the entire ingredients are melted.

Remove from heat and allow to cool for say 2 - 3 minutes.

Stir in flavor oil, vitamin E oil and a pinch of mica (optional)

Pour into lip balm tubes or lip tubes containers.

Leave untouched to solidify

Once set, it is ready for use.

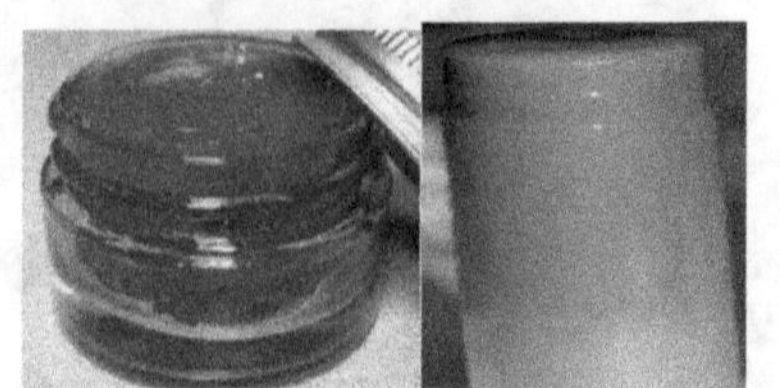

Honey Cinnamon lip

Ingredients

1 ½ tablespoon of beeswax

1 tablespoon of shea butter

2 teaspoon of coconut oil

1 teaspoon of apricot oil

1 teaspoon of honey

8 drops of cinnamon essential oil

Procedure

In a heat-safe bowl combine the beeswax, cocoa butter, shea butter, and apricot oil

Gently place on a pot of simmering water over medium-low heat.

Stir continually until the ingredients melt.

Remove the bowl from heat

Whisk in honey and cinnamon essential oil.

Pour in lip balm tubes or lip balm containers

Allow to solidify

Enjoy

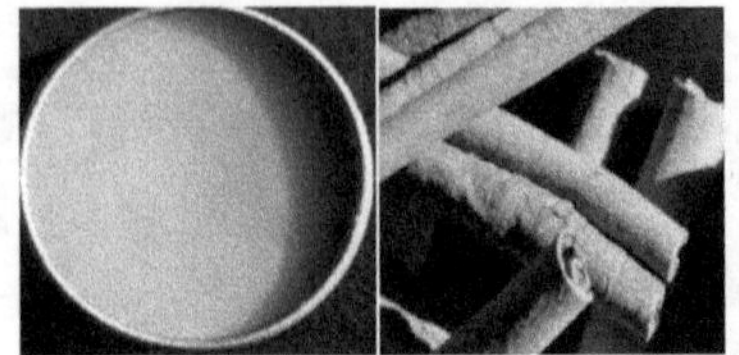

Coconut floral Balm

Ingredients

2 tablespoon of beeswax

2 tablespoon of virgin coconut oil

1 teaspoon of mimosa floral wax

1 and 1/2 tablespoon of cocoa butter

4 tablespoon of walnut oil

3 to 5 drops of Vitamin E oil

Procedure

In a double boiler, melt all the ingredients together over medium heat; stir till the entire ingredients are melted.

Transfer the mixture in the measuring cup.

Then pour inside the lip balm tubes or lip balm container

Allow for some time to cool. Once cool, it is ready for use.

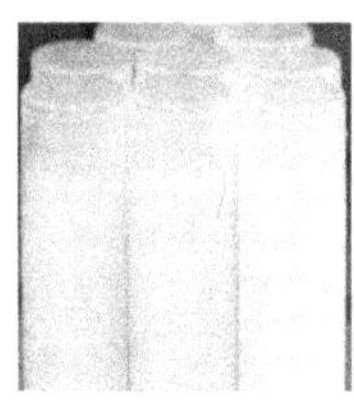

Maple syrup lip balm

Ingredients

5 g of beeswax

4 g of cocoa butter

3 g of virgin coconut oil

4 g of sweet almond oil

2 g of soy lecithin

4 g of dark maple syrup

Procedure

In a double boiler, combine the beeswax, cocoa butter, cocoa nut oil, almond oil, and soy lecithin.

Melt over medium heat; stir till the entire ingredients are melted.

Remove from heat.

Whisk in the dark maple syrup, continue whisking till the mixture cools and has reach room temperature.

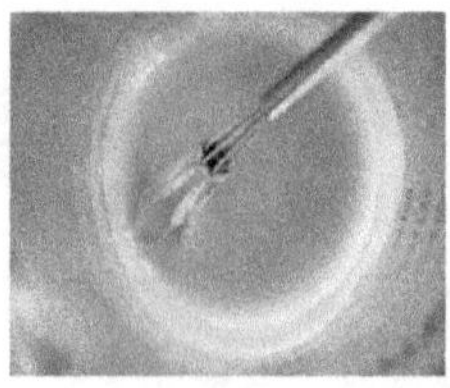

Use a spatula to scrap the emulsified mixture into lip balm containers.

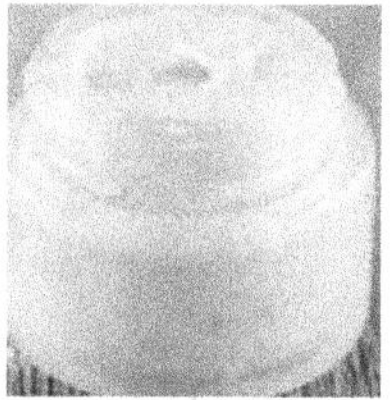

www.ingramcontent.com/pod-product-compliance
Lightning Source LLC
Chambersburg PA
CBHW070804250726
48662CB00004B/1974